Intermittent Fasting

The Unstoppable Intermittent Fasting Beginners Guide to Lose 3 Pounds of Fat a Week, Build Muscle, Stay Lean and Feel Healthier.

By

Beatrice Anahata

professional before attempting any techniques outlined in this book.

By reading this document, the reader agrees that under no circumstances are is the author responsible for any losses, direct or indirect, which are incurred as a result of the use of information contained within this document, including, but not limited to, —errors, omissions, or inaccuracies.

Table of Contents

Introduction 7

Why Fasting Diet Can Make You Burn More Fat ... 10

    1. Your Fat Burning Hormones are increased 10

    2. You have lots more fat burning enzymes 10

    3. You actually will burn more calories when
    fasting 11

    4. Instead of burning sugar you now burn more fat
    11

    5. You can understand what triggers you to eat. .. 12

    6. Get control back over what you eat. 12

    7. You can still enjoy all the foods you like. 12

Dietary and Exercise Considerations for Intermittent
Fasting 14

Weight Training Tips For Faster Weight Loss 18

    Muscle Metabolism Boost 19

    Proper Workout and Diet...................................... 19

    Post-Cardio Fat Burn 20

    Weight workout for fat loss 21

Changing Your Mindset 25

Choosing Your Exercise 26

Weight Lifting or Training....................................26

Don't overdo it 27

Set Goals 27

How to Incorporate Building Muscle During
Intermittent Fasting 28

Opt for training sessions that are scheduled late at
night..29

Consume the bulk of your caloric requirement after
your training session 30

Try to squeeze in a meal before 5 am 32

Does Exercise Play a Role in Intermittent Fasting?. 34

What Kind of Progress Should You See? 50

How Can You Track Your Progress?....................51

Weight Loss Effects 54

Preparing for and Preventing Setbacks 55

General Lifestyle Changes 58

Exercise 58

Water..59

Sleep 60

Nutrition 60

Conclusion...62

Introduction

When it comes to intermittent fasting, most people tend to think of fat loss. Believe it or not, intermittent fasting can also be an effective nutrition strategy for building muscle. Recall some of the benefits I mentioned earlier about fasting—specifically increased growth hormone and increased efficiency using fat for fuel.

The additional growth hormone will help you build more muscle, and you'll be less likely to store fat while you pack on muscle. So then what's the difference between fasting for fat loss and fasting to build muscle? The answer lies in a number of calories you need to eat. The caloric deficit is king for fat loss, and the caloric surplus is king for building muscle.

This means you must eat more calories than you burn off if you want to build muscle. Imagine you're an architect building a 2,600 square foot house. You'll need a certain number of bricks—say 6,000 for example—to build that house. If you don't have 6,000 bricks, then you'll have to downgrade the size of the house you're building.

Your muscles work the same way. If you want to build muscle, you must provide your body with enough of the raw materials (i.e. calories you get from food) necessary for it to happen. If you don't, then you'll be in the same boat as an architect without enough bricks. How many calories do you need to build muscle?

Use this simple equation:

Bodyweight in pounds x16=Daily caloric intake

Using myself as an example:

Bodyweight-195x16=3,120 calories

This means that I need to eat 3,120 calories every day to start gaining weight. One common complaint from guys is that they're a "hard gainer" or that they have a lightning fast metabolism. It doesn't matter how much they eat; they can't seem to gain any weight. The issue isn't that you're a hard gainer, it's the fact that you're not measuring how much you're eating.

You might think you eat a lot of calories, but until you track it how you will know? Simply put—you won't. The first thing you'll need to do is measure your weight. You have to know what your starting point is. From there, measure the number of calories in everything you eat and record it.

Use Google, My Fitness Pal, nutrition labels, and anything else you can to get an idea of how much you're eating. It'll never be exact, and that's ok. You want to get a rough measurement of how much you're eating. From there, track the calories in the note app on your phone.

This will be tough, but remember your mind, your goals and your strong determination will get you to your long-term goal. Let's go!!

Why Fasting Diet Can Make You Burn More Fat

Just to clarify when we talk about fasting diet what I mean is intermittent fasting where you only fast for 24 hours 2 or 3 times a week. This method is becoming a very popular way to help burn body fat in a short period and to help maintain your weight loss for life.

That said here are 7 ways this type of fasting can help you burn body fat quickly

1. Your Fat Burning Hormones are increased

HGH (Human Growth Hormone) is the most important fat hormone in our body. When we are a fasted state the production of this hormone is increased resulting in higher amounts of fat being burned. Fasting also allows the insulin levels in our body to reduce so you burn fat and not store it

2. You have lots more fat burning enzymes

When you are producing more fat burning hormones then you need a more fat burning enzymes to help them do their job properly. The two most important enzymes that assist in this process are Adipose tissue HSL and Muscle Tissue LPL. Simply explained the HSL

10

enzyme encourages your fat cells to release fat for energy to be used in your muscles and the LPL enzyme has the job of getting your muscles to soak up the fat so it can be burnt for fuel. Fasting increases the release of both these enzymes therefore creating a fantastic fat burning environment.

3. You actually will burn more calories when fasting

I have to admit I was not sure about this claim at first but after a few weeks of my fasting diet I found myself having extra energy and being more alert and awake on my fast days. The reason for this is that short term fasting (12-72hrs) actually boosts your metabolism and adrenaline levels. This combination results in extra calories being used and as we all know the more calories, you burn the faster you can lose weight.

4. Instead of burning sugar you now burn more fat

When you have a meal your body will first burn the carbs then the fat from your food. If you can't burn off this fat in few hours after this food then its going to be stored as fat. When you are fasting there is no other energy source in your body so it has to burn body fat and not the sugar in your blood put there by the food.

5. You can understand what triggers you to eat.

 When I made a decision to fast what surprised me most was how aware I became of the triggers and habits that made me eat badly. A lot of my unhealthy eating was down to routine and certain situations and by being able to see these more clearly, I started to break these bad habits. Knowing why and what causes you to eat certain foods is an important step to stopping this reaction can help build better habits.

6. Get control back over what you eat.

By doing short fasts, you do feel better about yourself and get a feeling of accomplishment. If you have issues with food then this positive response can help you build a positive relationship with food again. Being in control of what you eat will make sure you are not as vulnerable to eating all the bad foods that cause to put on weight.

7. You can still enjoy all the foods you like.

Short term fasting allows you to burn fat and ultimately lose weight while still enjoying foods you like. The discipline of fasting means on the other days you can have the foods you enjoy but without the guilt and still lose weight.

With this type of freedom in your diet you are far more likely to stick to the plan because you don't feel restricted. Most people fail to hit their goals because they stop too soon, so being able to be consistent over time is the difference between failure and success.

Dietary and Exercise Considerations for Intermittent Fasting

How will your diet affect your weight loss goals while practicing intermittent fasting?

The weight loss benefit of practicing this kind of cycled eating comes from not only stimulating your metabolism and other bodily processes through fasting but simply from having less time to consume as many calories as you would during a normal day. Most people tend to snack throughout the day, eat at least three large meals, and may even consume calories at night through snacks or drinks. By putting a limit on the length of time that calories are to be taken in, most people will drastically reduce the total number of calories per day. Grazing is a term used to describe the pattern of eating that many women find themselves doing, whether they know it or not. Unrestricted access to food is common in today's culture and is putting you at great risk for over consumption of calories—leading to continued weight gain. If you're someone who is used to this style of constant snacking and unrestricted eating, your body has grown accustomed to being fed all day long. This leads to a continual sensation of hunger and the urge to eat at all times throughout the day, rather than just at meal times. It can take some time to retrain your body and brain to limit hunger signals to the appropriate times of the day. Sticking to your intermittent fasting eating pattern will continue to feel easier each time you complete a fasting cycle.

If you have a normal diet, meaning you eat an average amount of food and don't partake in routinely binge or overeating, you should notice weight loss benefits from intermittent fasting without making changes to the foods you eat. This is one of the greatest perks of following the intermittent fasting "diet"! For many women, a diet has traditionally involved restricting calories for an extended period. Not only is this method of weight loss difficult to stick to—limiting the percentage of those who comply long term—but when you extendedly restrict calories, you create a reliance on high-quality nutrition as well. This is a major hang-up for many people who don't have the time to consistently prepare varied and nutritionally dense meals multiple times per day, as well as for those who are just unfamiliar with nutritional science and nutrient needs. Counting calories doesn't take into account the interactions within the body that are specific to every person and their diet. It can lead to a preoccupation with tracking foods consumed versus calories spent, creating mental stress and anguish—a contributing factor to the stalling of weight loss!

By following an intermittent fasting protocol, you don't have to worry about tracking how many calories you consume and logging your exercise to determine how many you've expended. You don't have to swear off your favorite snack foods, and you don't have to restrict yourself to only consuming nutritionally dense foods that you don't have to prepare or that you just don't like. Following your normal diet but planning it around specific hours will jumpstart your metabolism and ultimately provide the weight loss you've been looking for. Intermittent fasting cycling simplifies dieting and weight loss so that everyone and anyone can lose weight! You don't have to worry about preparing and cooking specialty health foods, purchasing overpriced supplements or meal replacements, or spending hours obsessing over certain foods and denying yourself your favorite snacks and treats.

If you find that during your periods of eating you tend to take in a large amount of junk food or you tend to overcompensate for your periods of fasting, you may want to consider making a few dietary changes to help you lose more weight quickly. While intermittent fasting simplifies dieting by eliminating the need to count calories and follow a strict dieting plan, consuming far too many calories will not provide weight loss. It is a simplified, effective weight loss tool, but it is not a magic solution to eating anything and everything you want in great quantity and lose weight! There is no magic solution, and if a diet program ever promises to be one, you should run the other way as fast as you can! It is a understood concept that too many calories in and not enough calories expended will not lead to weight loss, and depending on the difference between the two can even lead to weight gain. Even with the increase in resting metabolic function from the act of fasting intermittently won't completely negate an abnormally high-calorie diet during the non-fasting hours. When you first begin your intermittent fasting cycle, it may be helpful to keep an eye on the kinds of foods you're consuming during your "normal" days and your non-fasting periods, as well as the quantity. If you feel you may be overeating during these times or choosing mainly high-calorie foods, you can consider making a few dietary changes to fully benefit from the effects of your intermittent fasting cycles.

While not required, you may choose to make changes to your diet to experience the most benefits from intermittent fasting in the shortest amount of time. There are no specific nutritional requirements that the intermittent fasting protocol relies on, but a general focus on foods that are less processed can increase the quality of your calories and result in faster and speedier weight loss.

Weight Training Tips For Faster Weight Loss

You live a fit lifestyle year-round yet sometimes we realize the occasional junk food begins to demonstrate its effects. Being the educated fitness diva, you know it's time to start dieting and cook your workout to achieve your goal.

Be that as it may, for reasons unknown when you decide it's time to lose fat, the first thing we tend to do is bounce onto cardio, and weight training is not prioritized.

Whether this is on the grounds that the calorie-burning advantages aren't recognized, you think weight training is to build muscle and not burn fat, you think you can't focus on lifting and losing fat in the meantime, you don't know how to do an efficient weight training program, or whatever the reason. Some way or another we tend to return the weights on the rack when we want to focus on losing fat.

Although there are many benefits of cardio for fat loss, this article covers the advantages of using various weight training programs to lose fat.

You can never outrun a bad diet with just exercise; therefore, it is necessary to control diet as well in some instances. Exercises themselves have a great effect on your weight loss in the long run. There are two ways how this can go:

• Exercise more and eat even more, which will result in gaining weight instead of losing it.

• Exercise moderately and carry on with your diet and you will have an accelerated weight loss.

Muscle Metabolism Boost

First off, you ought to know what you've probably heard ordinarily: "Muscle burns fat." In any case, what does that mean? All things considered, muscle doesn't exactly burn fat, however, all the more precisely muscle raises your Resting Metabolic Rate (RMR).

Adipose tissue (i.e. fat) takes no energy to sit on your body, that is the reason once it's there it will stay there until you exert enough energy to start utilizing it as your energy source. Skeletal muscle tissue is called "active tissue" since it requires energy to maintain itself. To simply sit on your body, every pound of muscle on your body uses around 30-60 calories per day.

Proper Workout and Diet

With the right eating routine and workout, each one is capable of putting on 5 pounds of muscle in a year. If we estimate that your metabolism would utilize 50

19

calories per day to sustain that muscle, this means you will burn 250 more calories consistently (50 calories/day x 5 pounds). With a pound of fat requiring you to burn 3,500 calories, you will lose 26 pounds in a year without spending an additional moment on cardio. ([250 calories/day x 365 days/yr]/3,500 calories/pound of fat).

Presently as being stressed over fitness, sometimes we brush off this advice since we would prefer not to get "big" or "bulky." Our general public is acquainted with the amount of 5 pounds of fat is. We perceive how our bodies change when we gain or lose 5 pounds of fat. What is unfamiliar to us is the thing that 5 pounds of muscle is. Muscle is substantially more dense than fat.

At most gyms, the trainers have a copy of 5 pounds of fat and 5 pounds of muscle. I encourage you to ask a trainer that works there or the front desk person if you could investigate it. You'll be surprised by the volume difference, and you will see there is no need to worry about adding 5 pounds of muscle.

Post-Cardio Fat Burn

That hour of cardio was great to burn that stored energy, yet when you're done on the cardio machine, you're done burning calories. Weight training, then again, keeps your metabolism at an elevated energy use rate for 60 minutes after you're done. Another bonus to weight training!

Exercise science calls this afterburn effect Excess Post-exercise Oxygen Consumption (EPOC). This means after weight training the body continues to need oxygen at a higher rate.

Weight workout for fat loss

Hit it heavy

Muscle tissue growth is just empowered when pressure is applied to it. If you utilize light weights and do rep after rep, your muscle will never have the stress applied to it that it needs to respond as well. This means although you eat cleaner and are on a reduced-calorie eat less, your muscles won't grow.

Numerous dieters lighten up on their weight since they feel heavy is needed just during a bulking phase, and female dieters particularly would prefer not to lift heavy for fear of getting bigger rather than littler. These are myths no doubt.

Ladies should not shy far from heavier weights because they do not have enough testosterone to get the physique of a bodybuilder.

Lower rep/heavy weight workouts burn more calories during the workout due to greater exertion and will guarantee you won't lose an ounce of precious fat-burning muscle.

This workout uses mostly free weights since machines are designed to target individual muscle groups. This reduces the total amount of muscle required for moving the weight. The exercises will be mostly compound to recruit more muscle fibers to work and discharge muscle building and fat-burning hormones. Likewise, stay on your feet rather than sitting or lying down for whatever number exercises as would be prudent.

Speed it up

Doing higher reps with moderate weight could be beneficial for several reasons with regards to fat loss. The muscle fibers utilized during high reps are slow-twitch muscle fibers. These hold less glycogen; therefore less glycogen will be depleted from the body during the workout. This is critical for keeping the muscles full and the metabolism high.

Additionally, the increased lactate from high-rep training supports growth hormone (GH) output which is likewise a key hormone for losing fat.

Slow-twitch fibers likewise recover faster between sets than quick twitch fibers. This will make it possible for adherence to utilizing shorter rest intervals, and keep the heart rate up throughout the workout; thus burning more amounts of fat.

The same concept of utilizing mostly free weights and compound exercises as the heavy weight workout likewise applies to the lower-weight, high-rep workout above. Therefore, the same exercises can be applied however the weight needs to be adjusted to take into consideration more sets and reps.

Opt for Circuit Training

Circuit training is a half, and half kind of interval training where anaerobic (lifting) is combined with aerobic (cardio) exercise, using higher reps and lighter weights.

In your daily circuit you will do one set on a machine, then move to do a set on another machine, and on like that 'till you finish the circuit, bounce on a cardio machine for 10 minutes, and come back to your first machine, with no rest in between.

Anaerobic and aerobic exercise each provides their own particular unique physiological benefits. A unique advantage that circuit training has is it combines both. Quick twitch muscles are used primarily in anaerobic explosive exercises, while slow-twitch muscles are used primarily in aerobic endurance exercises.

One thing to keep in mind is that you'll use no less than two machines at a time. Keep in mind to be courteous at the gym and just do circuit training during off hours. Gym edict does not permit you to claim more than one station while other individuals are wanting to get through their workout also.

Double Up

Training muscles twice every week benefits from more regular training as well as the split lets you focus on intensity variation. Meaning, the first workout in the week will emphasize heavier weights and fewer reps while the second workout in the week will focus on moderate weight and higher reps.

Go for Supersets

The superset is a super-intensity technique for fat loss and muscle building. With these, you simply do two exercises back to back with no rest in between.

There are several reasons why supersets are more effective than doing the regular one station at a time with rests in between every set.

First, supersets increase Lactic Acid production. Additionally, supersetting is time efficient. By doing sets back to back you reduce your total workout time while as yet doing the same amount of work.

Supersetting involves doing two exercises with no rest in between.

In conclusion, different superset combinations can increase muscle fiber activation. This means you can utilize specific exercise combinations to increase the intensity of work on a specific muscle, helping it develop faster.

Changing Your Mindset

Never aim to lose extra weight by just and making a target of losing certain pounds in your schedules week or month as such approach never works when you are aiming to do exercise on a long-term basis.

Instead, go for exercise to gain more muscle mass and also feel better about yourself overall. As for the fat-losing part, let your diet cover you in the regard.

Don't think of exercising as a formality, do it for your pleasure and to gain confidence in yourself. Focus completely on your diet plan as it is a more important factor in losing weight than hitting the gym. Exercise in such cases is a boost to your weight loss campaign and also a way to keep you away from weakness as a result of weight loss.

Choosing Your Exercise

Lifting and high-intensity intermittent training are the most effective tools for weight loss on the long-term, especially when you are on a meal plan. You will know about both of them in this section.

Weight Lifting or Training

While doing your weight lifting with a trainer, try to focus on your major muscles and never forget about squats. Most of the diets have an effect called 'muscle-sparing effect' which will greatly help you preserve and build lean muscle mass further.

Putting on muscles is not as easy as most of the people think it is, it needs a lot of determination and courage to keep yourself on the same timetable for a long time. Weight lifting will offer you some assistance with building and keep up muscles and burn more calories while resting, as compared to how you did previously. It's a myth that you will develop huge muscles if you lift weights. It takes many years of workout to reach that level.

High-intensity Intermittent Training (HIIT)

This is also called interval running or training. It's a training method in which you interchange intense blasts of anaerobic exercise - for example, sprinting with short recuperation periods. One of the impacts is that you smolder more calories in less time contrasted with other workout schedules, such as delayed cardio.

Don't overdo it

You should exercise regularly, but make sure not to overdo it. Take rest days in between with sufficient sleep to meet your demands. Exercising more than your body is capable will increase the risk of getting injured. Furthermore, it will also negatively affect the immune system and increase hormones that are related to physiological stress, leaving you with more harm than good.

Set Goals

Always set your weight loss goals more than you think you can achieve and for that you will have to work out harder than you did before. You should always aim to lose more than 2 to 3 pounds per week.

If you are using a calorie calculator during your diet plan, do not go for large calorie deficits but try to settle ideally for no more than 500 Kcal and also depending on your basal metabolic rate (BMR) and activity level, shoot for a reasonable energy intake of 1300 to 1700 Kcal.

How to Incorporate Building Muscle During Intermittent Fasting

In recent years, many people have become curious about Intermittent Fasting. There may be a variety of reasons for this increasing interest. These reasons range from wanting to lose fat the easy way, to peoples' busy lifestyles. Many have no inclination to cook multiple meals a day. Some people also have busy schedules where they are unable to squeeze in a lunch or breakfast.

In some cases, Intermittent Fasting is followed by people due to certain beliefs. For example, by Muslims when they fast during Ramadan or otherwise from about 5 am to 7 pm.

Whatever your reasons may be, you may have wondered how you can build up any muscle mass while following this eating schedule. A lot of people assume that it is next to impossible to gain muscle mass while fasting. The fact is that if you spend a little time to plan out your day and your meals in the correct way, you can easily build muscles while fasting!

Here are some of the things that you should keep in mind to maximize your success.

Opt for training sessions that are scheduled late at night

If you are fasting for a specific period where you will be fasting from a set time in the morning to a set time in the evening (for example the Ramadan fasting set up of 5 am to 7 pm), it is best if you place your workout sessions for after 7 pm, as waking up and working out before 5 am will be a Herculean task.

It is always advisable that you consume some food before you start with your resistance-training program, so doing your training session before 7 pm is extremely unlikely. You also need to consume a certain amount of carbohydrates and proteins after your training program is over so that your body can begin the recovery process. You will not be able to do this if you are supposed to be fasting for that particular period.

When you start with a late evening training session, you can make sure that you consume your dinner immediately once you are home from work or as soon as your fasting period ends. This meal can act as a "pre-fuel" before you begin working out.

You can then start your training session, once you are done eating, say at around 7:30 pm and continue training for an hour or however long your workout lasts, giving you time to finish it by say 9 pm. This will give you enough time to squeeze a post workout meal into your schedule until it is time for bed at around 10 pm.

Consume the bulk of your caloric requirement after your training session

The second most important thing for you to do while following this protocol is to be sure that you consume the bulk of your required caloric intake immediately after you finish working out. As mentioned before, this post workout meal helps the body with regeneration. By helping the body to recover from the workout, this post workout meal aids in the generation of lean muscle mass in the body.

For this to work, you first need to figure out the number of calories that you need to consume in a day so that you can build up an adequate amount of muscle mass. Once you figure out your total caloric needs for the day, consume about 20% of the required calories right before you begin working out. This meal should contain both carbohydrates and proteins, as this meal will act as a fuel for your workout. If you do not consume adequate carbs or proteins, you will feel extremely lethargic and tired.

After you finish your daily workout, the post workout meal should consist of about 60% of your total required calories. These calories can also be divided into 2 or 3 small meals in the time span that ranges from post work out to bedtime.

This meal is likely to contain a large number of calories that you need to consume in a short span of time. You may find it difficult to consume the required quantity of calories all together. It helps to focus on consuming foods that have a large number of calories, such as red meat, dried fruit, bagels, raw oats, etc.

You should also keep in mind that the meal you are consuming is immediately after you finish working out. So, with this kind of a meal plan set up, you should consume high carb foods that will help in building muscle, rather than opting for foods that are high fat and low carb. This is because immediately after working out, your body requires carbohydrates. In this scenario, if you provide your body with more fat, it will have a detrimental effect on your body.

This doesn't mean that you have to eliminate all the fat from your diet. You can consume a meal that has a lot of carbs or proteins just after you finish your training and then consume a high fat or high protein meal just before you sleep. The point is to keep the fat consumption low in the meal that immediately follows the workout session.

Fatty foods are more calorie-dense, and it is extremely easy to eat them in a large amount, for example, nuts, butter, oils, etc. These are easier to consume than a lot of high carb foods – especially when you are already feeling satiated. So, it is best if fatty foods are consumed as a second small meal just before bed, while carbs are consumed immediately after working out.

Try to squeeze in a meal before 5 am

The last thing that you need to do while following this approach to building muscle while Intermittent Fasting is to eat a meal immediately after you wake up. For all of the people who aren't following Ramadan and are just fasting to lose weight/gain muscle mass, this meal can be consumed at whatever time you naturally wake up.

If you are following Ramadan, it is advisable that you wake up earlier, say around 4:30 am, just before the fast begins, and consume a slow digesting protein, such as red meat with some cottage cheese, that will make up for the remaining 20% calories that you need to consume.

You can also add in some fat or carbs to this meal, but make sure that you consume about 35% of your required protein at this time. This ensures that there is a steady supply of amino acids in the body while you fast throughout the day.

After consuming the meal, you can go back to sleep if you want.

Make sure that when you follow this type of muscle building Intermittent Fasting regimen, that you keep all of the points above in mind. If you try to perform a large volume of highly intense exercise while consuming very few calories, your body will react negatively to it, and you will do yourself more harm than good.

Slowly, the body will lose all the stored glycogen and will be deprived of it. This will result in lethargy, the inability to keep up with your workouts and the incapability to recover. To be sure that this doesn't happen to you, you will need to force feed yourself until your body becomes acclimated to this meal cycle. Eventually, this approach will start feeling normal to you and your body.

Does Exercise Play a Role in Intermittent Fasting?

As promised, intermittent fasting will produce weight loss for most women regardless of the incorporation of an exercise regimen. Pairing your intermittent fasting cycle with a lifestyle that isn't sedentary will be enough. Not sitting for long periods of time and regular movement are both important factors in any healthy lifestyle and any diet routine aimed at weight loss.

Regular movement and even exercise can be an important aspect of any weight loss plan, but exercise alone won't cancel out continuously poor dietary choices. The foods you consume have a greater impact on the regulation of weight than does your physical activity or fitness.

So, the bottom line is that most women don't need to exercise to lose weight while practicing intermittent fasting, but if you want to incorporate structured exercise into your routine, certain activities can give you the most "bang for your buck." Plus, as an bonus, exercise can be a temporary appetite suppressor, and one study of overweight participants showed that those who engaged in physical activity every other day while following an intermittent fasting program lost more weight than the group that didn't.

The best exercise routine to pair with your intermittent fasting cycle is to visit the gym three times per week and perform a brief warm up, a weightlifting routine, and a few cool down and stretching poses. Now, I know what you're thinking. Don't be intimidated by the mention of exercise or weightlifting. As promised, the addition of regimented physical activity to your cycled eating is optional, and you may find you don't need or wish to incorporate it into your intermittent fasting practices. The beauty of this plan is in its universal effectiveness—it can benefit everyone from body builders to you!

For those who are interested in a workout routine that will optimize their weight loss while following an intermittent fasting eating plan, I've simplified the science behind these specific exercises as well as created an easy-to-follow regimen that will provide you with confidence at the gym. And of course, you don't need to worry about these weightlifting exercises making you appear bulky or muscular; they are specifically geared toward women's bodies and when combined with intermittent fasting, can help you achieve a toned, healthy look!

Lifting weights will burn calories while providing an extra boost to your metabolism (on top of the increased metabolic stimulation intermittent fasting provides.). Studies have shown that even while actively following a diet plan and losing weight, weightlifting can build muscle.

Rules for incorporating simple exercise into your intermittent fasting weight loss routine:

• On the days you are fasting, do a light physical activity like yoga, low-intensity swimming, or light cardio like a brisk walk or slow jog.

• On the days you are not fasting, do a more intense physical activity like high-intensity interval training or weight lifting.

•Drink plenty of water when doing physical activity, on fasting and non-fasting days!

An example of a high-intensity interval training exercise can be as simple as follows:

Three rounds: 20 seconds of exercise and 10 seconds of rest between each exercise.

1.   Air boxing: Stand with your right foot slightly in front of your left and your hips pointed toward your left side. Set your arms in a boxer's stance and punch with your right arm toward your left side, and then punch with your left arm headed toward your right side. Repeat.

2.   Air boxing (again): Rotate your stance so that your left foot is slightly in front of your right and your hips point toward your right side. Again, take your boxer's stance and punch with your left arm first followed by your right.

3.   Jumping jacks: Simply do as many jumping jacks as you can do in the 20 seconds of allotted time.

4.   Squats: Do as many squats as you can in the 20 seconds of allotted time, ensuring you are squatting deep enough to feel your thigh muscles begin to tire.

An example of a simple weight training routine for women:

A weight lifting routine for women does not have to be complicated, heavy, or produce bulky results. Engaging your muscles in weight lifting activity will keep your bones strong and healthy, lower your risks of osteoarthritis, and build muscle mass, thus increasing the speed of your metabolism and providing you with the toned arms and legs that most women seek. Weight lifting does not always have to include lifting actual weights! Bodyweight exercises are incredibly effective for slightly increasing a woman's muscle mass and shaping her body.

Always warm up before beginning your routine!

Start by doing squats. Try doing somewhere between 8 and 12 squats, take a small rest, and repeat one more time.

Use one light dumbbell in each hand (approximately 8 pounds) to do two sets of rows, somewhere between 8 and 12 rows per set. Stand with your feet apart, in line with your knees, and your knees slightly bent. Keep your back flat and lean forward from your hips. Lift the weights up to your chest while pulling your shoulders back. Your elbows should be bent and pointed backward while your palms face in.

Next, use your body weight to do push-ups. Start out doing them on your knees, and move to a full push-up whenever you feel capable. Again, do two sets of 8 to 12 push-ups, increasing the number as you gain strength and are able.

Finally, end your routine with a plank. To do this, you'll hold your chest off the floor with your forearms, while your toes face the floor. Lower your waist toward the floor until your body becomes a straight line, parallel to the floor. Start by holding this position for as long as you can, eventually working your way up to a 60-second hold.

Don't be intimidated by the incorporation of exercise into your intermittent fasting routine. Increasing your physical activity will benefit your weight loss and provide an even greater boost of energy. Don't feel that you need to start everything at once! You may find it easier to begin your fasting routine for a few weeks before you add in an exercise routine. The most important aspect of any weight loss program is to do what works for you! This will increase the likelihood that you'll stick with it long enough to see results.

What to do about low energy?

Low energy is one of the hardest hurdles to overcome (other than hunger) when you're on an IF diet. The biggest reason for this is that there are many different causes. With hunger, there are defined reasons you could be hungry. Ghrelin and several psychological cues all cause hunger. So what causes low energy? It could be hundreds of different physical factors. So, instead of focusing on what causes hunger, let's jump right into solutions. These solutions include seeing your doctor for bloodwork in case you're low on vital nutrients, exercise, taking a shower, meditation, napping, going outside, and switching your IF method.

Seeing Your Doctor

The first thing that you should do when you're too tired while fasting is to see your doctor. It's very important to rule out a physical cause before moving onto something like exercising. It's not necessary to see a specialist; just your local friendly GP will do. You may want to call ahead of time and check that they've worked with patients on special diets before. Not all doctors will be familiar with the benefits of IF.

After you've found a doctor to see, make an appointment that's most convenient for you. In the time between your appointment and now it may be best to take a break from your fast if you are feeling unwell. Your health should always come first.

On the day of the appointment, your doctor will ask you a lot of questions about your diet. Make sure you come prepared with your medical history, and all of the details of your diet prepared. Your doctor will most likely prescribe some amount of blood work or supplements. They may even suggest some of the things you've already read this book! Your doctor is your partner in your weight loss/health journey, so it's critical that you follow their advice. Be sure to ask your doctor whether or not you can continue your fast while you wait for your test results if he or she has ordered them.

Once the test results are back, your doctor or a nurse may call you back with your results. They may ask you to come back for a follow-up appointment. If your fatigue is explainable by the results of your blood work, your doctor will work with you on a solution suited to your situation.

Exercise

There are many types of exercise out there, but the benefits are all the same - improved health, strength, and the benefit of natural endorphins. Exercise is also proven to provide a natural boost to your energy level. For this reason, IF and exercise usually go hand in hand. However, certain types of heavy exercise that require a lot of energy (calories) should probably be avoided while on a fast. For example, you probably shouldn't run a cross country marathon while also fasting! Here are four great examples of exercise that works well with fasting.

Running

There are hundreds of books, articles, and websites dedicated to the benefits of running. Unless you suffer from a severe medical illness, there are no downsides to running. There are even some anthropologists who argue that the human body was built for long distance running. In fact, some hunting tribes in Africa simply outrun their prey. The prey eventually becomes too tired to escape!

One of the best programs for a beginning runner is called "Couch to 5k". It is free to use and requires no special equipment. You simply run three times a week using a special timed schedule, especially for beginners. The first week's three sessions all start with a 5-minute walk. Then, 60 seconds of jogging. Finally, 90 seconds of rest. Repeat for 20 minutes. That may seem easy to handle, but if you're just starting out, you may be surprised at its difficulty. You can read about the full program on Cool Running's website, coolrunning.com.

The benefits of running to focus and attention were shown in a study by scientists at the University of Illinois in 2003. Twenty men were tested using a device on their heads that measured brain activity. They were measured before and after 30 minutes on the treadmill with mental tests. The areas of the brain known to contribute to focus and attention were significantly more active after the run. You can use these same benefits to your advantage while you fast!

Yoga

Yoga is a mental exercise as much as it is a physical one. It originated in India around the sixth or fifth century BCE. Back then, Yoga was mostly a religious practice. It's come a long way since its origins. Now everyone around the world participates in Yoga for its many benefits. It has a very spiritual core to its practice, but you don't have to believe in anything to try it and experience its benefits. It's been shown to lower risk of heart disease as well as help to energize those who practice it.

The best way to start yoga is to get hands on teaching from a local "yogi" or teacher. They're pretty easy to find through the internet these days - just search "yoga practice [your city here]." You'll get many results!

Another way to start yoga is by doing it yourself at home. You can look up beginner poses online, or even watch videos on popular websites like YouTube that will guide you through everything you need to do. It's best, to begin with small 15 to 20-minute total body yoga sequences before moving onto anything advanced. All you need to begin is a mat. Even a towel will work if you don't have a yoga mat.

It's best to perform your yoga practice at the same time every day. You could even dedicate a certain space in your home or workplace for this purpose.

Swimming

There's nothing quite like jumping into a cold pool of water to wake you up! This, combined with exercise is a great way to wake yourself up if you're feeling fatigued. To top it off, it's cheap! All you need is a local pool and a swimsuit. If you don't already know how to swim, there are many classes offered at local recreation centers. This exercise is best used in the morning or evenings after work. There are many advantages to swimming over another exercise.

Water makes you highly buoyant. When you are submerged up to your neck, you are 90% buoyant. That means that exercise is much easier. You won't hit the floor quite as hard, and you'll have increased flexibility. There's also constant resistance from the water all around you. There's an estimated 12 to 14% more resistance in water than on land. That means you'll be working harder for the same amount of exercise than you would do on land. Lastly, water is great for keeping cool. This makes it a great option if you hate getting sweaty and hot when you exercise.

Besides swimming laps, there are a lot of water exercise options including:

1. Water walking: simply walk in neck deep water.

2. Water aerobics: exercises performed to increase the heart rate for 20 minutes or more.

3. Water strength training: using water exercise equipment, such as floaters, to increase resistance and strength.

4. Flexibility training: increasing your range of motion through stretching.

5. Water Yoga: yoga designed to be performed in a pool of water.

6. Deep water running: simulates running on land with special flotation devices.

Each of these exercises, or even just lap swimming, will increase wakefulness and help fight fatigue.

Dance

Dance is exercise and also my personal favorite! It's particularly good at taking your mind off any stress you might have because you have to coordinate movements and focus. Many exercise classes today even incorporate dance. Ever heard of Zumba? How about Jazzercise? These are two of many types of exercises popular these days that heavily incorporates dance. Dancing is an efficient way to bring your heart rate up, have fun, and get some great cardio in as well. Whether or not you think you can dance well, the movement will be enough to wake you up.

Your first, easiest, and cheapest option is to turn on the tunes and get into the groove simply. You can do this by yourself, or with others if you're confident enough! Since it's only to wake yourself up, there's no reason to worry if you're doing it "right." Brushes make great impromptu microphones if you'd like to sing along.

Your second option is to take a dance class. Simply search online for dance classes near you. There will be many to choose from. These are some of the best types of dance to increase your alertness by raising your heart rate:

1. Zumba

2. Jazzercise

3. Swing dancing

4. Salsa dancing

5. Belly dancing

6. Pole dancing

If you still can't decide on a class, listen to the type of music that would be played in the class. Choose the class for which you like the music best. This will make the class more fun. Therefore you'll be more likely to keep going.

Showering

Showering is something you probably already do in the morning to wake yourself up. If you work from home or have access to a gym with a shower at work, this is a great quick option that you can use on your lunch break. You'll feel cleaner as well as being more alert. If you feel that a full shower would be too much to take, don't worry. You don't need to use soap, shampoo, conditioner, or anything else you normally do in the shower. This is purely for the purpose of waking up. To optimize your experience follow these steps:

1. Step into the shower, and turn on the water to a comfortable temperature.

2. Enjoy the warm water for 5 minutes.

3. After you're comfortable, turn the water to be as cold as you can take it for 30 seconds. The colder, the better. This step is important.

4. After your 30 seconds is up, turn the water to be as hot as you can take it for another 30 seconds. Again, the hotter, the better. This is also important. It will increase your blood flow and stimulate you further.

5. End the shower with one more 30-second bout of cold water. Again, as cold as you can stand it.

This is a form of something called "hot and cold hydrotherapy." It's been around for thousands of years. It reduces stress and increases your tolerance to stress. It strengthens your immune system. The cold water tightens your blood vessels, increasing your blood pressure which is fantastic for your heart's health. And last but not least, it will certainly wake you up!

Meditation

While it's great for focusing your mind on fighting hunger and cravings, it's also fantastic for helping you increase alertness and fight fatigue. This may seem like a bit of a paradox at first. How can something relaxing and calming cause you to feel more alert and awake? You'll be surprised to find out that there have been studies that prove meditation is a great tool for this purpose. More than that, meditation can help you mentally to cope with and become accustomed to your new IF diet.

Stress is a very large reason for why we become tired in the first place. Changing your lifestyle can be very stressful. For that reason, you'll probably be pretty tired when you start your IF diet. The part of your brain that is most active during stressful or tiring events is the amygdala. During mediation, the amygdala decreases its activity significantly. Meditation will help you to manage and maintain this benefit. Often, you may find that your stress was misplaced or based on fear the meditation will help you work through.

Another benefit of meditation is that it has no side effects like sugary energy drinks. Energy drinks, coffee, and supplements are very temporary solutions. And it's dangerous to drink too much in one day. They often leave you feeling more tired than you started afterward. Thankfully, meditation has no side effects! You meditate as much as you'd like with no negatives afterward. In fact, a chemical often used in energy drinks is DHEA. It has been proven that your body naturally produces more DHEA when you meditate. It's a great all natural alternative.

To feel more awake, it's important that you get good sleep. Meditation helps to increase the quality of your sleep. It will make you more mindful in your waking hours so that you go to bed on time and relaxed. This is important for your health in general, but especially while you are fasting and your body is burning its energy resources.

Going Outside

Going outside is a natural and easy option to help with fatigue. Light has been shown to assist with many sleep and mood disorders, such as seasonal depression and delayed sleep phase disorder. Sometimes these conditions are treated with special light equipment. However, all you need to increase wakefulness would be 10 to 20 minutes spent in the outdoors. Going outdoors to do some quick grocery shopping will take your mind off things and can easily add 1-2 hours to your fast.

What Kind of Progress Should You See?

As with any new eating or exercise regime, you can expect there will be some fluctuations throughout your week. While overall you can expect to lose 3-8% body weight (and a bit of your waist!) within your first 3-24 weeks, the important thing to remember is that there may be some up and down to start. However, over time, you should expect to see weight loss throughout your fast, no matter which type you've chosen. The weight loss should be steady, and while some fasts may cause you to lose more weight (because some fasts may cause you to lose muscle, as discussed), you should notice these effects no matter which fast you've chosen.

You should see a decrease in fat and an increase in muscle mass (unless you're doing an extended fast) once your body has normalized. Your clothes will fit differently, you will move differently, and your taste in food may even change as your pallet is cleansed through fasting.

After you've been on a fast for about a week or so, you should notice you aren't feeling as hungry as you used to. Your body has adapted to the new eating schedule, and you should be able to get through your fasts a little easier. In fact, your body will have stopped craving food at times it used to be accustomed to being fed at and now will crave food to the new schedule you have forced it into. This is great progress because it shows your body is adapting and it will then be easier on you to continue your fast.

Your mood will stabilize if you're at the right level of fasting for yourself — if it hasn't stabilized after about ten days, you will need to consider one of the options we discussed earlier: either change your fasting cycle by decreasing your fasting days or decrease your workout intensity.

There's a chance you may have to change what activities you do at what times. Perhaps you aren't focusing as well in the afternoon as you were before. Well, try to move those activities to the morning when you are more critically alert. You should notice increased clarity since you have simplified your eating routine and made the appropriate adjustments to decrease the negative effects of having too much fat on your body (lethargy, trouble focusing, etc.).

How Can You Track Your Progress?

Start by recording your weight before you start your plan, as well as your measurements. Take before photos. This combination is the best way to see your true success from home. If you have a gym membership or access to the coaching staff, you can ask them to help you with these things.

Your doctor can also help you with some important measurements like blood pressure, cholesterol levels, blood sugars, and other specific medical testing that cannot be done at home. If this interests you, then try to book in with your doctor about once a month to keep track of these measurements. These can be some of the better measures of your true health because they are internal factors that are directly influenced by diet and exercise, as opposed to strict body image (just because a person is thin, doesn't mean they're healthy inside; vice versa for someone who is very muscular).

Pick a day and a time that is consistent, week-to-week, to show your true results. As mentioned before, you may notice some fluctuations early on, but this baseline will help you realize the true effects later on. Not only that but if you see a 1-2-pound fluctuation in a week, that is nothing to be concerned about; in fact, that is quite normal.

As your fast goes on, you will now have a baseline and a consistent measurement schedule to help keep you focused and on track. It is important that you eliminate as many variables as possible, so you get the most accurate results possible.

Other, less scientific, ways to measure your progress is to keep track of how you feel each week, both regarding general feelings about the fasting, but also in regards to how you are feeling on a mental and physical level. Notice how your clothes fit differently as the weeks go by. Do you have a particular pair of pants or a shirt that is a little too tight or ill-fitting right now for you to feel comfortable in? Add it to your assessment each week and see how your body is adapting by how that article of clothing is starting to fit. Maybe you are increasing your muscle size, and you have a shirt you need to fill out more — this is the same situation: try it each week to see when it finally looks the way you want to. The pictures help a lot with this because as you go through each week, you can see physical changes you may not notice in the mirror. We look at ourselves a lot during a day, so the captured image of a photo can help us realize the differences when we put them side by side.

Energy levels may also change as you go through the process. They may go up and down as the weeks go on, so keep track of these, too. You may be able to problem solve some issues by reflecting on when you feel tired and how long your bouts of lethargy last. Sometimes caffeine will help you through these times if you find you're truly struggling, or perhaps even a nap. Napping may help get you through some of your cravings and provide you with a mental boost as well.

Weight Loss Effects

Surprisingly, there are positives and negatives associated with losing weight. We have discussed many of the positives already, but some of the negative side effects can be things like loose skin, seeing stretch marks that you didn't notice before, having to buy all-new clothes (this can be an expensive task!), and having to adjust certain medications that depend on hormone and weight balance.

These negative effects can often be offset by patience, determination, and your doctor's assistance. Once you've figured out that living a healthy, fit life is well-worth these potential setbacks, you will overcome any obstacles set in your path and embrace the new you.

You will likely have more energy and feel more confident than you had before. Your workouts will get more complicated and fun, and you'll notice you're capable of more types of activity than before. With some coaching or personal training assistance, or by doing a ton of research and hopefully getting experienced feedback from someone who knows how to workout properly, you will be able to try new exercises in and out of the gym. This will help you overcome any potential stagnation that can happen when your body adjusts and creates a new homeostasis that you need to work past.

When you lose healthy amounts of weight, you become more trim and fit. You may find yourself open to new experiences like zip lining or scuba diving that you didn't feel confident trying before. Perhaps you'll join that sports team you wanted to but never felt fit enough for. The confidence you will feel by representing your best self, through your hard work and determination will show through when you have adjusted to your transformation. Wear that outfit, try that activity, be competitive with yourself for your personal best in running or lifting.

Preparing for and Preventing Setbacks

Inevitably, you are going to run into obstacles. Some of them are going to throw you off course — sorry, but it is bound to happen! Life is going on around you, and it could throw you a curveball like an unexpected pregnancy (whether yourself or your partner) or a vacation opportunity that prevents you from eating as you had planned. Even if something like this happens, there are some steps you can do to prepare for and prevent some of these setbacks.

Have a backup plan: you may have your heart set on a specific fasting plan, but keep a backup ready just in case. If you are getting off track regularly, the plan you've chosen isn't working for you, instead try your backup plan! Have your reasons ready for why you can't join in a night of drinking, or have that treat. Your friends and family will respect your decisions, and likely appreciate the head's up that you are fasting! You know, just in case you are moody.

Don't put yourself in situations that you know might tempt you until your fast is over. If you know your best friend's birthday is coming up, but you want to do an extended fast, make sure that you have enough time to do your fast and recover from it before that day. Otherwise, have your backup plan ready to go! Try to minimize that kryptonite food you have lying around the house, even now. Are you a chips person? Or maybe a cookie monster? Make it, so you have to consciously plan and act to get these favorite snacks so you are less likely to do so. This will protect your fasting plan and also your waistline.

Plan early and plan often. If you start with a well-rounded plan for your meals and your workouts, you have a better chance of succeeding. Plan them out as far in advance as possible, so you don't have to worry about last minute adjustments — or, worse, so you don't get stuck when you lose your motivation to workout or stick to your fasting regime. Whether this entails planning detailed meals each day for your plan, scheduling your workout and fasting times appropriately, or even creating workout programs for yourself for the duration of your fast, you are in control of every step you take. It may help you to plan all these things, or at least sketch them out so that you don't put yourself in a situation where you have to use your backup plan as your main plan!

Ask for help. Again, tell your family and friends what you are planning to do. If you have a partner, while you shouldn't expect anyone to join you in this endeavor unless he or she wants to, you can ask them to help you through the worst times. Maybe they can do more meal prep, so you don't have to work with food if you're struggling with your fast. Perhaps they can plan your re-feed days with an exciting dinner out together to celebrate your success. If all else fails, they're a sympathetic ear when the going gets tough.

General Lifestyle Changes

When you decide to add fasting to your way of life, the first thing to remember is that you need a healthy lifestyle. That means including all of the elements included in this chapter. If you do not include them already, then now is the time to start. You will find fasting quite hard if any of these elements are missing from your life, so use these as a springboard because they are necessary.

Exercise

We live in a very sedentary society. That's why a lot of people have weight and mobility problems. In our household, for example, my husband and I were average overweight people whose lives were busy but did not encourage exercise. My husband's mobility problems started years ago, and when we decided to exercise, we took it slowly at first, walking around the yard several times and then increasing that gradually. Don't tell me you can't do it. We were probably the most unfit people you can imagine, and we managed to do it. You have to move the body, or you will find that it's too hard to move out of your chair. Even if you can't do strenuous exercise, start small. Then, we started swimming, and that's a wonderful exercise because it also teaches you to breathe in the right way. There are all kinds of exercises that you can do that are fun and exercise doesn't have to be the dirty word that the public is making it.

If you have a dog, that's a good reason to go for a walk. If you are housebound, you can still exercise because exercise can be done anywhere and these days there are so many apps available that you can even exercise in the privacy of your own home. You need to know that exercise helps you to distribute the food that you eat to the right places in the body and if you simply sit and eat, all of that food will turn into fat.

Water

Drinking water is essential if you are thinking of going into fasting. You should be drinking up to 8 glasses a day, and many people just don't do that. Let's take a look at what water drinking does. Water helps with the transportation of all the nutrients in the food that you eat to all the different areas of the body. It helps to keep your body hydrated, and although you may not put a lot of value on that, let's try and show you what happens when you don't drink sufficient water. Waste and bacteria in the body are not flushed out. There is the risk of illnesses such as colon cancer. Apart from these, the body needs water to keep inflammation at bay, and if you are trying to lose weight by fasting, water is essential. Raw fruit and vegetables also contain water so are helping you to get some water into your system, but if you seriously want to use a detox fasting system, water is vital to the picture. Get used to drinking water and lots of it, but glass by glass, rather than gulping it down in a couple of sessions. You need to have water throughout the day so always carry a bottle with you and if you don't like the taste of it, use flavorings such as a slice of lemon and even make water into green tea for some of the time.

Sleep

You need eight hours sleep a night. If you are unhealthy and want to fast, then you will need all the help you can get from nature. Sleep is nature's way to heal the body and if you deprive yourself of sleep, don't expect to stay on a fast for a long time because you will fail. There are other reasons for wanting to sleep for 8 hours. During the fasting, those eight hours is helping you to pass the fasting period without even thinking about it. That's very valuable indeed if you want to do the fast work for you.

Nutrition

It makes sense that if you were to fast for a period and then eat fifteen bagels, you would still retain the weight that you said you wanted to lose. Be honest with yourself while you are fasting. Fasting isn't a fad. It's a lifestyle choice. You have chosen this lifestyle because you want to lose weight. Although you have a license to enjoy foods, there is a really little point in even trying if you can't be sensible about your food choices. You need to eat a variety of fruits and vegetables and avoid all of those high sugar, high carb foods that you know to be bad for you. Your body needs a certain amount of carbs, but you need to balance out your eating so that you enjoy it but so that it is nutritionally sound as well. I say this because you have to remember that I come from a family of "fatties" and I know all the tricks in the book as far as cheating is concerned. When you cheat, the only person being cheated is yourself.

Conclusion

We have come to the end of the book. Thank you for reading and congratulations for reading until the end.

I hope the book has opened your eyes to the endless ways through which you can lose 3 pounds of fat a week, build muscle, stay lean and feel healthier.